# The AFib Diet for Seniors

A Heart-Healthy Guide with Age-Friendly Recipes & a 3-Week Plan to Manage Atrial Fibrillation

copyright © 2025 Isadora Kwon

All rights reserved No part of this book may be reproduced, or stored in a retrieval system, or transmitted in any form or by any means, electronic, mechanical, photocopying, recording, or otherwise, without express written permission of the publisher.

# Disclaimer

By reading this disclaimer, you are accepting the terms of the disclaimer in full. If you disagree with this disclaimer, please do not read the guide.

All of the content within this guide is provided for informational and educational purposes only, and should not be accepted as independent medical or other professional advice. The author is not a doctor, physician, nurse, mental health provider, or registered nutritionist/dietician. Therefore, using and reading this guide does not establish any form of a physician-patient relationship.

Always consult with a physician or another qualified health provider with any issues or questions you might have regarding any sort of medical condition. Do not ever disregard any qualified professional medical advice or delay seeking that advice because of anything you have read in this guide. The information in this guide is not intended to be any sort of medical advice and should not be used in lieu of any medical advice by a licensed and qualified medical professional.

The information in this guide has been compiled from a variety of known sources. However, the author cannot attest to or guarantee the accuracy of each source and thus should not be held liable for any errors or omissions.

You acknowledge that the publisher of this guide will not be held liable for any loss or damage of any kind incurred as a result of this guide or the reliance on any information provided within this guide. You acknowledge and agree that you assume all risk and responsibility for any action you undertake in response to the information in this guide.

Using this guide does not guarantee any particular result (e.g., weight loss or a cure). By reading this guide, you acknowledge that there are no guarantees to any specific outcome or results you can expect.

All product names, diet plans, or names used in this guide are for identification purposes only and are the property of their respective owners. The use of these names does not imply endorsement. All other trademarks cited herein are the property of their respective owners.

Where applicable, this guide is not intended to be a substitute for the original work of this diet plan and is, at most, a supplement to the original work for this diet plan and never a direct substitute. This guide is a personal expression of the facts of that diet plan.

Where applicable, persons shown in the cover images are stock photography models and the publisher has obtained the rights to use the images through license agreements with third-party stock image companies.

# Table of Contents

**Introduction**     7
**Atrial Fibrillation and Aging–What Seniors Need to Know**     9
    How Aging Affects the Heart and Circulation     9
    Common AFib Symptoms in Seniors vs. Younger Adults     11
    Medication, Lifestyle, and Diet: Finding the Right Balance     12
    Key Nutrients for Heart Health as You Age     14
**The AFib-Friendly Diet for Seniors**     15
    Heart-Healthy Foods to Embrace     15
    Foods That May Trigger AFib Episodes     17
    The Importance of Hydration and Electrolyte Balance in Older Adults     18
    Adapting Portion Sizes and Nutrient Needs for Seniors     19
**Meal Planning Made Simple for Seniors**     22
    Creating Balanced, Easy-to-Digest Meals     22
    Meal Timing and How It Affects AFib Symptoms     23
    Grocery Shopping Tips for Seniors (Budget-Friendly and Low-Prep Options)     23
    How to Adjust Meals for Common Senior Health Concerns (Diabetes, Arthritis, High Blood Pressure)     29
**Gentle Cooking Methods for Heart Health**     31
    Easy-to-Chew & Digestible Cooking Tips for Older Adults     31
    Reducing Sodium Without Sacrificing Flavor     33
    Safe Cooking Strategies for Those with Limited Mobility or Dexterity Issues     34
**Age-Friendly Recipes for AFib Management**     37
    Breakfasts: Simple, Nutritious Morning Meals     38
    Lunches & Dinners: Low-Sodium, High-Nutrient Comfort Foods     44
    Heart-Healthy Snacks: Quick Bites for Energy & Stability     52
    Desserts: Sweet Treats Without the Sugar Overload     56

| | |
|---|---|
| **The 3-Week AFib Action Plan for Seniors** | **61** |
| Week 1: Small Tweaks for Big Impact | 61 |
| Week 2: Building a Sustainable Routine | 67 |
| Week 3: Lifestyle Habits for Long-Term Heart Health | 73 |
| **Beyond Diet – Lifestyle Tips for Senior AFib Management** | **79** |
| Managing Stress and Anxiety for a Calmer Heart | 79 |
| The Role of Light Exercise and Safe Physical Activity | 81 |
| Sleep and AFib: How to Improve Rest as You Age | 88 |
| How to Talk to Your Doctor About Diet and Medication Interactions | 89 |
| **Conclusion** | **92** |
| **FAQs** | **94** |
| **References and Helpful Links** | **97** |

# Introduction

Atrial fibrillation (AFib) is a type of irregular heartbeat that can seriously impact your quality of life, especially as you age. AFib becomes more common in seniors because the heart naturally undergoes changes over time.

For example, the heart muscles might become less elastic, affecting their ability to pump blood efficiently. This decline often happens alongside age-related conditions like high blood pressure, diabetes, or arthritis, making AFib management more challenging for older adults.

Unlike younger adults, seniors may experience AFib symptoms more subtly. While some feel heart palpitations or a racing pulse, others might mostly notice fatigue or shortness of breath. Understanding these differences is the first step to effectively managing the condition.

While medication is often a core part of managing AFib, diet can be just as important. The food you eat can help regulate your body's electrolyte balance, reduce inflammation, and even lower your risk of stroke. For seniors, eating well isn't just about addressing AFib. It's about meeting the unique nutritional needs that come with aging.

A thoughtful diet tailored to manage AFib focuses on eating nutrient-rich whole foods, staying hydrated, and avoiding processed ingredients or known triggers like excess salt or caffeine. Adjustments to portion sizes and the incorporation of key nutrients like potassium and magnesium can provide extra benefits.

In this guide, we will talk about the following:

- Atrial Fibrillation and Aging – What Seniors Need to Know
- The AFib-Friendly Diet for Seniors
- Meal Planning Made Simple for Seniors
- Gentle Cooking Methods for Heart Health
- Age-Friendly Recipes for AFib Management
- The 3-Week AFib Action Plan for Seniors
- Beyond Diet – Lifestyle Tips for Senior AFib Management

Keep reading to learn more about how you can take control of your AFib and enjoy a healthy, fulfilling life. By the end of this guide, you'll have the tools and knowledge to create a personalized dietary plan that works for you.

# Atrial Fibrillation and Aging–What Seniors Need to Know

## How Aging Affects the Heart and Circulation

The aging process causes several natural changes in the heart and blood vessels that can impact overall cardiovascular health and increase the risk of conditions like atrial fibrillation (AFib). Understanding these changes is vital for managing AFib effectively.

1. **Heart Stiffness and Function**

    As you age, the walls of the heart can become thicker and stiffer. This reduces its flexibility and makes it harder for your heart to fill and pump blood efficiently. Over time, this can lead to a condition known as diastolic dysfunction, a common contributor to AFib in seniors.

2. **Electrical Changes in the Heart**

   Your heart's natural electrical system, which controls its rhythm, can begin to lose efficiency. Aging may lead to slower signal transmission or misfires, resulting in irregular heartbeats or arrhythmias like AFib.

3. **Arteries Narrowing and Losing Elasticity**

   With age, your arteries may harden or narrow due to a buildup of plaque, a condition called atherosclerosis. This increases blood pressure and forces your heart to work harder, elevating the risk of AFib and other heart-related complications.

4. **Decreased Resilience**

   Older hearts have a reduced ability to recover from stress, such as illness or physical exertion. This leaves seniors more vulnerable to conditions like AFib when the body is under strain.

Combined, these issues can lead to reduced heart function, higher blood pressure, and a greater likelihood of episodes of AFib. Staying proactive with lifestyle changes, medications, and a heart-healthy diet is essential to counteracting these age-related challenges.

# Common AFib Symptoms in Seniors vs. Younger Adults

The symptoms of AFib can vary widely between seniors and younger individuals. Seniors often experience different or more subtle symptoms, which may go unnoticed or be mistaken for other health issues.

## Common Symptoms in Seniors

1. *Fatigue and Weakness*: Seniors often report feeling unusually tired or weak, which may be attributed to slower heart rates or poor circulation caused by AFib.
2. *Shortness of Breath*: This often occurs even without physical activity and may mistakenly be seen as a result of age or lack of fitness.
3. *Dizziness or Lightheadedness*: AFib can reduce blood flow to the brain, leading to episodes of dizziness, which may raise concerns about falling risks.
4. *Chest Discomfort*: Some seniors experience vague sensations in the chest, such as tightness or mild discomfort, rather than the palpitations commonly felt by younger individuals.

## Differences from Younger Adults

Younger people with AFib often feel more pronounced palpitations or a racing heart, which can prompt quick diagnosis. Seniors, on the other hand, may not notice these signs or may attribute them to other common aging concerns, such as stress or fatigue.

For seniors, symptoms like tiredness, breathlessness, or lightheadedness can easily be misinterpreted as general signs of aging. If you or a loved one experiences any of these, it's important to consult a doctor for evaluation.

## Medication, Lifestyle, and Diet: Finding the Right Balance

Effectively managing AFib requires a tailored balance of medication, lifestyle adjustments, and dietary choices. Here's how these elements interact and support each other:

1. **The Role of Medications**

   Medications are often the first step in managing AFib, but they aren't a stand-alone solution. Regular check-ups are important to ensure the medications are working effectively and not causing side effects. **Common AFib medications include:**

   - *Blood Thinners*: Prevent blood clots and reduce the risk of stroke.
   - *Rate Control Medications*: Help keep your heart rate within a safe range.
   - *Rhythm Control Medications*: Work to restore or maintain a normal heartbeat.

2. **The Importance of a Healthy Lifestyle**

   Pairing medications with a heart-conscious lifestyle can strengthen their effectiveness. This includes:

   - *Exercise*: Low-impact activities like walking, swimming, or yoga improve heart health without overexerting it.
   - *Stress Management*: AFib episodes can be triggered by stress, so incorporating relaxing activities is crucial. Techniques like meditation, journaling, or spending time with loved ones can help calm your heart.

3. **How Diet Complements Treatment**
   - A balanced, nutrient-rich diet can reduce AFib triggers, improve circulation, and lower related risk factors like high blood pressure or weight gain. Limiting caffeine, avoiding added sugars, and reducing alcohol consumption can dramatically reduce AFib episodes.
   - Aim to include plenty of heart-healthy foods while working closely with your doctor to identify potential interactions between medications and certain foods.

**Practical Tip:** Use a meal tracker to document how your AFib fluctuates in response to your diet. This will help you and your doctor identify effective habits or foods to avoid.

## Key Nutrients for Heart Health as You Age

To age well with AFib, focus on foods rich in these key nutrients for heart health:

- *Omega-3 fatty acids*: Found in fatty fish like salmon, these healthy fats reduce inflammation and stabilize your heartbeat.
- *Potassium*: Crucial for balancing blood pressure; bananas, oranges, and spinach are great sources.
- *Magnesium*: Supports healthy muscle and nerve function, including the heart. Look for dark leafy greens, nuts, and seeds.
- *Fiber*: Helps control cholesterol and blood sugar, reducing strain on the heart. Oats, beans, and fruits are excellent sources.
- *Antioxidants*: Found in brightly colored fruits and vegetables, antioxidants help prevent cell damage and support overall heart health.

Making sure your diet includes these nutrients while avoiding processed foods high in salt, sugar, or unhealthy fats is key to heart health.

# The AFib-Friendly Diet for Seniors

An AFib-friendly diet plays a crucial role in managing symptoms and supporting heart health, especially for seniors. With proper planning, dietary adjustments can reduce triggers, stabilize heart rhythms, and improve overall well-being. This chapter outlines the key components of such a diet and provides practical guidance tailored to seniors.

## Heart-Healthy Foods to Embrace

Eating a diet full of nutritious, whole foods can help seniors manage AFib and keep their hearts healthy. Here are some key food groups to include in daily meals:

1. **Fruits and Vegetables**

   Fruits and veggies are loaded with vitamins, minerals, and antioxidants that protect the heart. Leafy greens like spinach and kale provide potassium and magnesium, which help keep the heart's rhythm steady. Bright options like berries, oranges, and carrots add even more heart-friendly nutrients. Seniors should aim for 4–5 servings of fresh or frozen fruits and vegetables every day.

2. **Whole Grains**

Whole grains like oats, quinoa, brown rice, and whole-grain bread are high in fiber, which helps lower cholesterol and keeps blood vessels healthy. Swapping out refined grains for whole grains can also provide longer-lasting energy.

3. **Lean Proteins**

Good protein choices include skinless chicken, fish rich in omega-3s (like salmon and mackerel), and plant-based options like beans, lentils, and tofu. These proteins help maintain muscle without putting extra strain on the heart. Omega-3s, in particular, can reduce inflammation and support a steady heart rhythm.

4. **Healthy Fats**

Healthy fats from foods like avocados, nuts, seeds, and olive oil can lower bad cholesterol and improve heart health. Omega-3-rich foods also help reduce the risk of irregular heartbeats. Use olive oil instead of butter or other saturated fats for cooking.

5. **Low-Fat Dairy**

   Low-fat dairy products like yogurt and milk provide calcium and potassium, which are good for the heart, without the extra saturated fat. Look for fortified, low-sodium options to maximize the benefits.

By focusing on these heart-healthy foods, seniors can create meals that help control blood pressure, provide essential nutrients, and reduce inflammation—key factors in managing AFib.

## Foods That May Trigger AFib Episodes

Certain foods and beverages can trigger or worsen AFib symptoms by disrupting heart rhythm, causing inflammation, or increasing blood pressure. Seniors should be aware of these triggers and limit or eliminate them from their diets:

1. *Caffeine:* Excess caffeine from coffee, tea, energy drinks, or chocolate may stimulate the heart and trigger irregular rhythms. Though moderate intake is generally safe, seniors with AFib should monitor their sensitivity and limit consumption to a maximum of one cup per day.
2. *Alcohol:* Alcohol, especially in large amounts, can disrupt the heart's electrical signals and increase the frequency of AFib episodes. Even small amounts can act as a catalyst, so seniors should consider avoiding alcohol entirely or limiting intake to special occasions.

3. ***High-Sodium Foods:*** Sodium can elevate blood pressure, placing extra strain on the heart. Avoid processed snacks, frozen meals, canned soups, and salted condiments. Look for "low-sodium" or "no added salt" alternatives and aim to keep daily sodium intake below 1,500 mg.
4. ***Processed and Sugary Foods:*** These foods are often high in unhealthy fats, sodium, and sugar, which increase blood pressure and inflammation. Packaged snacks, baked goods, and sugary beverages should be replaced with healthier alternatives like nuts, seeds, or fresh fruit.

By identifying and avoiding these triggers, seniors can significantly decrease the likelihood of experiencing AFib episodes and better manage their overall condition.

## The Importance of Hydration and Electrolyte Balance in Older Adults

Proper hydration and electrolyte balance are essential for heart health, particularly in seniors. Dehydration can disrupt the body's normal electrolyte levels and cause heartbeat irregularities, escalating the risk of AFib episodes.

1. ***The Role of Electrolytes:*** Electrolytes like potassium, magnesium, and sodium are crucial for maintaining normal heart rhythm. A deficiency or imbalance in

these nutrients can weaken the heart's electrical signals, leading to arrhythmias.
2. *Staying Hydrated:* Seniors should aim for 6–8 cups of water daily unless otherwise advised by their doctor due to medical conditions like kidney disease. Those who find plain water unappealing can add slices of lemon, cucumber, or berries for flavor.
3. *Managing Electrolytes:* Incorporate potassium-rich foods such as bananas, spinach, and sweet potatoes, and include magnesium sources like almonds and legumes. Coconut water is another hydrating option loaded with electrolytes but should be consumed in moderation to avoid excessive sugar.
4. *Practical Tips for Seniors:* Keeping a water bottle nearby serves as a simple reminder to hydrate. During hot weather or illness, fluids should be increased to prevent dehydration-related complications.

Maintaining proper hydration and electrolyte levels helps protect the heart's rhythm and supports overall cardiovascular health, making it a critical component of an AFib-friendly diet.

## Adapting Portion Sizes and Nutrient Needs for Seniors

Aging affects the body's ability to process and absorb nutrients, making portion sizes and balanced meals even more important. Seniors should adjust their diets to accommodate these changes while still meeting their heart health goals.

1. ***Changes in Metabolism:*** With age, the metabolism slows down, meaning the body requires fewer calories but still needs the same amount of nutrients. This makes it essential to prioritize nutrient-dense foods while controlling portion sizes to avoid overconsumption.
2. ***Balancing Meals:*** Each meal should include a mix of lean protein, whole grains, and colorful vegetables. For example, a balanced plate might consist of grilled chicken, quinoa, and a side of sautéed spinach. Opt for smaller but frequent meals to maintain steady energy and avoid overeating.
3. ***Practical Strategies:*** Invest in smaller plates to encourage appropriate portion sizes. Pre-portion snacks like nuts or pre-sliced fruit to make healthy choices easier. Avoid skipping meals, as this can lead to overeating later on or triggering AFib symptoms.
4. ***Addressing Specific Nutritional Needs:*** Seniors may require additional calcium or vitamin D to support bone health or need softer foods for easier digestion. Fortified cereals, low-fat dairy, and high-fiber vegetables should be included to meet these needs without compromising heart health.

By adapting portion sizes and focusing on nutrient-rich foods, seniors can create a diet that supports their changing nutritional needs while promoting better management of AFib.

An AFib-friendly diet for seniors centers on minimizing triggers and maximizing heart-healthy foods in their daily meals. With careful planning and consistent effort, dietary changes can help reduce episodes, stabilize rhythms, and enhance long-term quality of life.

# Meal Planning Made Simple for Seniors

Now that we have a better understanding of the key principles behind an AFib-friendly diet, let's explore some practical tips and strategies for meal planning. This will help seniors make healthier choices and avoid common pitfalls when it comes to their daily meals.

## Creating Balanced, Easy-to-Digest Meals

When planning meals, the key is balance and simplicity. Seniors may have unique dietary needs, including the necessity for foods that are gentle on the stomach. A balanced meal should include lean protein (like chicken, fish, or beans), whole grains (such as brown rice or quinoa), and plenty of vegetables. Healthy fats, like olive oil or avocado, can also be included in moderation.

For easy digestion, consider cooking methods like steaming, baking, or simmering. For example, a meal of steamed fish, roasted sweet potatoes, and sautéed spinach is packed with heart-friendly nutrients while being simple and light on the stomach. Aim for smaller portion sizes if large meals feel overwhelming and avoid too much fiber in one sitting, which can sometimes cause discomfort.

## Meal Timing and How It Affects AFib Symptoms

The timing of your meals can impact your energy levels and even contribute to managing AFib symptoms. Focus on eating smaller meals throughout the day rather than heavy ones, which can put stress on the body. Avoid eating too close to bedtime, as lying down with a full stomach may increase acid reflux, potentially triggering AFib.

For seniors, regular meal times help maintain blood sugar stability and energy. A good routine might be breakfast around 8 AM, a light lunch around noon, a healthy snack at 3 PM, and dinner by 6 PM. Listening to your body's signals is important, so avoid skipping meals, as this can lead to low energy levels and affect your heart rhythm.

## Grocery Shopping Tips for Seniors (Budget-Friendly and Low-Prep Options)

Shopping for heart-healthy meals doesn't have to feel overwhelming or break the bank. With a little planning and some strategic choices, you can fill your pantry with nutritious ingredients that are easy to prepare and kind to your heart. Here are some expanded tips to make your grocery trips both efficient and budget-friendly:

1. **Plan Ahead with a Versatile Grocery List**

   Before heading to the store, write down a list of staples that can be used in several meals. This saves time, reduces waste, and ensures you always have healthy options on hand. Some versatile items to include are:

   - *Whole grains* like brown rice, quinoa, or oats. These can form the base of your meals, like breakfast porridge, grain bowls, or side dishes.
   - *Dry or canned (no-salt) beans* such as lentils, chickpeas, and black beans. They're great for soups, salads, and side dishes.
   - *Frozen fruits and vegetables* like berries, spinach, or broccoli. These last longer than fresh produce and are already prepped, saving time.
   - *Healthy pantry staples* like olive oil, vinegars, and unsweetened almond milk for cooking and dressings.

   Consider planning weekly meals before shopping. For example, if you're making quinoa as a side on day one, you can use leftovers in a salad or soup later in the week. This reduces food waste and makes cooking easier.

2. **Choose Fresh or Frozen Produce Over Canned**

   Fresh and frozen produce are excellent choices for seniors managing AFib. Fresh fruits and vegetables are bursting with nutrients and flavors, while frozen produce offers convenience and a longer shelf life.

   Why avoid canned goods? Many canned options contain added sodium or preservatives that aren't heart-friendly. If you do need to buy canned items, look for varieties labeled "no salt added" and rinse them under water before use to reduce sodium content further.

   - *Shop seasonally*: Seasonal produce typically costs less and tastes better. For instance, apples and squash are affordable in the fall, while berries are best in the summer.
   - *Pro tip*: Visit your local farmer's market for fresh, affordable produce whenever possible. Many markets offer discounts toward the end of the day.

3. **Buy in Bulk When Possible**

   Bulk purchases can save you money and ensure you're stocked up on nutritious staples. Focus on items with a long shelf life, such as:

   - *Nuts and seeds*: Walnuts and flaxseeds are heart-healthy options loaded with omega-3 fats.

Store them in airtight containers or the fridge to keep them fresh.
- *Whole grains*: Bulk bags of rice, oats, or barley can be portioned into reusable containers for easy access.
- *Legumes*: Dried beans and lentils are less expensive than canned options and can be soaked and cooked in batches to use throughout the week.

Many grocery stores have bulk sections where you can measure only as much as you need, making this a great option for seniors managing smaller households or budgets.

## 4. Simplify Protein Choices

Protein is essential for a balanced diet, but it doesn't have to be expensive. Focus on affordable, heart-healthy options like:

- *Eggs*: A budget-friendly choice that's easy to cook and very versatile. Enjoy them scrambled, boiled, or turned into heart-healthy veggie omelets.
- *Canned fish*: Tuna, salmon, or sardines are rich in omega-3 fatty acids. Always opt for low-sodium varieties packed in water rather than oil.

- ***Lean meats***: Look for smaller cuts of lean chicken or turkey, which can be stretched across multiple meals by adding veggies or grains.
- ***Other options***: Tofu or tempeh are plant-based, protein-packed alternatives that are often budget-friendly and adaptable to several cuisines.

Consider batch-cooking and freezing portions of lean proteins, like baking several chicken breasts at once, so you can defrost and use them as needed.

5. **Time-Saving Pre-Prep Options**

Many stores offer pre-prepped ingredients that can make cooking easier, especially for seniors with limited energy or mobility. While they may cost slightly more, they're still cheaper and healthier than eating out.

- ***Pre-chopped vegetables***: Save time on dicing onions, carrots, or celery, ideal for soups and stir-fries.
- ***Steamed-ready bags***: Look for microwaveable bags of frozen vegetables that can be prepared in minutes.
- ***Cooked grains***: Some supermarkets offer pre-cooked quinoa, rice, or farro in individual pouches for quick meals.

For those on a tighter budget, an afternoon spent chopping, roasting, or steaming fresh produce in advance can achieve similar convenience.

6. **Take Advantage of Discounts and Loyalty Programs**

Many grocery stores offer senior discounts, loyalty cards, or weekly promotions. Take a few minutes to check weekly flyers or digital coupons for deals on items you already plan to buy, like fresh produce, frozen veggies, or pantry staples.

- *Look for deals on perishable items*: Many stores mark down fresh produce or meats nearing expiration. If you find a deal, you can freeze items like chicken or berries for later use.
- *Compare brands*: Store-brand items are often much cheaper and just as nutritious as their name-brand counterparts.

7. **Don't Shop When Hungry**

A simple but essential tip for sticking to a heart-healthy budget is to avoid shopping on an empty stomach. Hunger can lead to impulse purchases, often of less nutritious, packaged snacks. Eat a light meal or snack before heading to the store so you can focus on your list and budget.

8. **Use Grocery Delivery Services**

   If mobility or transportation is a concern, grocery delivery can reduce stress and save time. Many stores offer affordable home delivery services or curbside pick-up options, allowing you to shop online and avoid carrying heavy items. Check for local services or apps that can compare prices for you.

By following these tips, grocery shopping for a heart-healthy AFib-friendly lifestyle can become budget-friendly, stress-free, and nutritious. Preparing ahead and making thoughtful choices will not only save money but also simplify your meal planning weekly!

## How to Adjust Meals for Common Senior Health Concerns (Diabetes, Arthritis, High Blood Pressure)

Meal planning should not only be heart-friendly but also take into account other common senior health concerns. Here's a quick summary of meal adjustments for these conditions.

1. **Diabetes**
   - Focus on meals rich in fiber and low-glycemic foods, such as oatmeal, lentils, or non-starchy vegetables.

- *Example Meals*: A turkey and vegetable stir-fry with quinoa or a salad with grilled chicken and avocado.

2. **Arthritis**
   - Include anti-inflammatory foods like fatty fish, leafy greens, and berries.
   - Avoid processed items or foods with trans fats that can worsen inflammation. A sample meal is baked salmon with roasted sweet potatoes and steamed spinach.

3. **High Blood Pressure**
   - Reduce sodium intake by avoiding salty snacks and seasoning with herbs instead of salt.
   - Add potassium-rich foods like bananas or yogurt to balance blood pressure. Example Meal: Grilled chicken with a side of avocado salad and roasted zucchini.

By tailoring meals to these health concerns, seniors can manage not just AFib, but also other conditions commonly associated with aging.

Planning meals doesn't have to be complicated or time-consuming. By choosing simple, balanced meals, eating at regular intervals, shopping for smart options, and addressing specific health concerns, seniors can maintain both heart health and overall well-being with ease.

# Gentle Cooking Methods for Heart Health

Cooking in ways that prioritize heart health doesn't have to be complicated. Gentle preparation methods can make meals easier to chew and digest, enhance flavor without extra salt, and accommodate physical challenges that some seniors may face. This chapter provides practical cooking tips tailored for seniors managing AFib while addressing other needs.

## Easy-to-Chew & Digestible Cooking Tips for Older Adults

Many seniors benefit from meals that are not only healthy but also easy to chew and digest. Preparing food in ways that soften textures and support digestion can make eating more enjoyable and manageable.

1. **Opt for Gentle Cooking Techniques**
   - *Steaming*: This method preserves nutrients while softening vegetables like carrots, broccoli, or zucchini without overcooking.

- *Slow-Cooking*: Slow cookers are ideal for creating tender meals like stews or soups with ingredients such as lean meats, lentils, and vegetables.
- **Baking or Roasting**: Gentle roasting at moderate temperatures can enhance flavors while keeping foods tender. For example, bake fish or roast sweet potatoes until soft.

2. **Puree or Mash When Needed**

For those with difficulty chewing, pureeing soups or mashing vegetables like potatoes and squash can make meals more suitable. Smoothies made with fruits, yogurt, and oats are also easy-to-consume options.

3. **Choose Soft Proteins**
   - Incorporate tender proteins like baked fish, ground turkey, or scrambled eggs. Plant-based proteins like tofu and beans are also soft and easy to digest.
   - If using tougher cuts of meat, cook them slowly in broth or sauce to achieve a melt-in-the-mouth texture.

4. **Avoid Hard or Crunchy Foods**

Limit items like raw carrots, nuts, or crackers unless they are softened with cooking or paired with dips like hummus or avocado.

By using gentle techniques and choosing soft ingredients, seniors can prepare meals that are nutritious, easy to enjoy, and kind to their digestive systems.

## Reducing Sodium Without Sacrificing Flavor

Reducing sodium is crucial for managing heart health, but it doesn't mean meals have to taste bland. Using natural flavor enhancers and seasoning creatively can elevate dishes while supporting low-sodium diets.

1. **Experiment with Herbs and Spices**
   - Replace salt with fresh herbs like parsley, basil, rosemary, or cilantro. Spices like cumin, smoked paprika, or turmeric can bring depth to dishes without added sodium.
   - For a zesty punch, sprinkle lemon zest or squeeze fresh lime over meals.
2. **Infuse Flavor Naturally**
   - Cook grains like rice or quinoa in unsalted broth or infuse water with garlic, onion, or bay leaves during preparation.
   - Marinate proteins in mixtures of olive oil, vinegar, garlic, and herbs for added taste before cooking.
3. **Use Low-Sodium Alternatives**
   - Opt for reduced-sodium or "no-salt-added" canned goods and condiments. For instance, try

- low-sodium soy sauce or homemade salad dressings instead of store-bought ones.
- Nutritional yeast is another option for adding a cheesy flavor without salt.

4. **Create Seasoning Blends**

   Combine your own salt-free blends using spices like garlic powder, onion powder, paprika, and dried thyme. For example, a mix of smoked paprika, black pepper, cumin, and oregano works well on chicken or roasted vegetables.

These small changes can lower sodium levels dramatically while keeping meals satisfying and full of flavor.

# Safe Cooking Strategies for Those with Limited Mobility or Dexterity Issues

Cooking can present challenges for seniors with arthritis, decreased grip strength, or mobility issues. Adaptive tools and thoughtful planning can make meal preparation safer and more efficient.

1. **Invest in Adaptive Kitchen Tools**
   - Use utensils with large, soft-grip handles for easy holding, such as ergonomic vegetable peelers or spatulas.
   - Electric can openers, jar openers, and lightweight pots and pans can prevent strain on

joints. Food processors and choppers simplify chopping tasks.

2. **Prioritize Stability and Safety**
   - Place a non-slip mat under cutting boards or bowls to prevent sliding during meal prep.
   - Use knives with ergonomic handles and keep them sharp to minimize the pressure needed to cut ingredients.

3. **Simplify Meal Prep**
   - Purchase pre-chopped vegetables or pre-cooked grains to save time and effort. Pre-packaged salad mixes and frozen fruits are also quick, healthy options.
   - Batch cook meals and freeze portions for easy reheating later. This reduces the need to cook daily.

4. **Use One-Pot or One-Pan Recipes**

   Simplify cooking by preparing meals in one pot or pan to reduce the number of dishes. Options like hearty stews, casseroles, or roasted sheet-pan meals are easy to manage and clean up.

5. **Opt for Countertop Appliances**

   Small appliances like slow cookers, air fryers, and microwaves are senior-friendly and reduce the need to stand for long periods in front of a stove.

By incorporating these tools and strategies, seniors with physical limitations can safely prepare meals that meet their nutritional needs.

Gentle cooking methods contribute significantly to heart health and overall well-being. Preparing soft, easy-to-chew meals improves comfort and digestion, reducing sodium enhances flavor for better heart management, and adaptive tools make cooking accessible for all. Together, these strategies ensure that seniors can continue enjoying the process of creating and sharing healthy meals while managing AFib.

# Age-Friendly Recipes for AFib Management

Eating well to manage AFib doesn't have to be complicated or tasteless. This chapter is packed with age-friendly, heart-healthy recipes designed especially for seniors. These meals are easy to prepare, gentle on digestion, and packed with the nutrients your body needs to thrive.

# Breakfasts: Simple, Nutritious Morning Meals

### Banana Oatmeal with Chia Seeds

*Serves*: 1

*Preparation Time*: 10 minutes

### Ingredients:

- ½ cup rolled oats
- 1 cup unsweetened almond milk (or low-fat milk)
- ½ ripe banana, sliced
- 1 tablespoon chia seeds
- ¼ teaspoon cinnamon
- Optional toppings: walnuts, blueberries

### Instructions:

1. Combine the oats and almond milk in a small pot. Cook over medium heat, stirring occasionally, for about 5 minutes until thickened.
2. Add the sliced banana and chia seeds. Stir well to combine and cook for another 2–3 minutes.
3. Sprinkle with cinnamon and add optional toppings, like a handful of walnuts or a few fresh blueberries, for extra flavor and nutrients.

## Why It's Good for AFib

This filling breakfast provides potassium from the banana, omega-3s from chia seeds, and fiber from oats, all of which promote heart health and stable energy levels.

## Spinach and Mushroom Egg Scramble

*Serves*: 2

*Preparation Time*: 15 minutes

### Ingredients:

- 2 large eggs + 2 egg whites
- 1 teaspoon olive oil
- 1 cup fresh spinach
- ½ cup chopped mushrooms
- ¼ cup diced tomatoes
- Pinch of black pepper

### Instructions:

1. Heat olive oil in a non-stick skillet over medium heat. Add the mushrooms and sauté for 2–3 minutes until softened.
2. Toss in the spinach and tomatoes and cook for another 1–2 minutes until the spinach wilts.
3. Beat the eggs and egg whites together in a small bowl and pour them into the skillet. Stir gently until the eggs are cooked through.
4. Season with black pepper and serve with a slice of whole-grain toast.

## **Why It's Good for AFib**

This protein-rich scramble is low in sodium and packed with magnesium, fiber, and antioxidants from the vegetables, supporting your heart's overall health.

## Avocado and Tomato Whole-Grain Toast

*Serves*: 1

*Preparation Time*: 5 minutes

### Ingredients:

- 1 slice whole-grain bread, toasted
- ¼ ripe avocado
- 2 slices of tomato
- A dash of black pepper

### Instructions:

1. Mash the avocado with a fork and spread it evenly over the toasted bread.
2. Place the tomato slices on top and sprinkle with a little black pepper for seasoning.
3. Enjoy this simple and delicious breakfast right away!

### Why It's Good for AFib:

Avocados provide healthy fats and potassium, which supports heart health and reduces the risk of irregular heart rhythms. The whole-grain bread adds fiber for steady energy and balanced blood sugar levels.

# Berry Yogurt Smoothie

*Serves*: 1

*Preparation Time*: 5 minutes

## Ingredients:

- ½ cup plain low-fat Greek yogurt
- ½ cup mixed fresh or frozen berries (blueberries, strawberries, raspberries)
- ¼ cup unsweetened almond milk (or water)
- 1 teaspoon ground flaxseeds

## Instructions:

1. Combine the yogurt, berries, almond milk, and flaxseeds in a blender.
2. Blend until smooth and creamy.
3. Pour into a glass and enjoy this quick and refreshing morning treat!

## Why It's Good for AFib:

This smoothie is rich in heart-friendly nutrients, including omega-3s from the flaxseeds and antioxidants from the berries. The yogurt provides protein, while the almond milk adds calcium without unnecessary sodium or sugar.

# Lunches & Dinners: Low-Sodium, High-Nutrient Comfort Foods

## Lemon Herb Salmon with Steamed Broccoli

*Serves*: 2

*Preparation Time*: 20 minutes

### Ingredients:

- 2 salmon fillets (4–6 oz each)
- 1 tablespoon olive oil
- Juice of ½ lemon
- 1 teaspoon dried basil or dill
- 2 cups broccoli florets
- 1 cup cooked quinoa

### Instructions:

1. Preheat the oven to 375°F (190°C). Place the salmon fillets on a baking sheet lined with parchment paper.
2. Drizzle olive oil and lemon juice over the salmon and sprinkle with basil or dill. Bake for 12–15 minutes, until the salmon is flaky.
3. Steam the broccoli for 5–7 minutes, until tender but still bright green.
4. Serve the salmon and broccoli alongside cooked quinoa for a nutrient-packed meal.

## Why It's Good for AFib

Salmon is rich in omega-3 fatty acids, which help reduce inflammation and improve heart function. The quinoa and broccoli add fiber, magnesium, and antioxidants.

## Lentil and Vegetable Soup

*Serves*: 4–6

*Preparation Time*: 45 minutes

### Ingredients:

- 1 tablespoon olive oil
- 1 medium onion, diced
- 2 cloves garlic, minced
- 2 cups chopped carrots and celery
- 1 cup dried lentils, rinsed
- 6 cups low-sodium vegetable broth
- 1 teaspoon dried thyme
- 1 cup chopped spinach

### Instructions:

1. Heat olive oil in a large pot over medium heat. Sauté the onion and garlic until fragrant (about 3 minutes).
2. Add carrots, celery, lentils, vegetable broth, and thyme. Bring it all to a boil, then reduce the heat and simmer for 30–35 minutes, or until the lentils are tender.
3. Stir in the spinach during the last 5 minutes of cooking.
4. Serve warm with a sprinkle of fresh parsley.

## Why It's Good for AFib

This hearty soup is loaded with potassium and magnesium from the lentils and vegetables. It's warming, low in sodium, and perfect for digestion.

## Stuffed Bell Peppers with Quinoa and Veggies

*Serves*: 4

*Preparation Time*: 40 minutes

### Ingredients:

- 4 large bell peppers (any color)
- 1 cup cooked quinoa
- 1 cup chopped tomatoes
- ½ cup diced zucchini
- ¼ cup diced onion
- 1 tablespoon olive oil
- 1 teaspoon dried oregano
- ½ cup shredded low-sodium mozzarella or plant-based cheese (optional)

### Instructions:

1. Preheat the oven to 375°F (190°C), prepare bell peppers by slicing off tops and removing seeds, then place upright in a baking dish.
2. Cook onion, zucchini, and tomatoes in olive oil, then add quinoa and oregano.
3. Spoon the quinoa mixture into the hollow bell peppers. Top with cheese if desired.
4. Bake for 25–30 minutes, until the peppers are tender and the tops are slightly golden.

5. Serve each stuffed pepper warm for a wholesome, colorful meal.

**Why It's Good for AFib:**

Bell peppers are rich in antioxidants, while quinoa provides magnesium and fiber. This dish is satisfying, low in sodium, and packed with heart-healthy ingredients.

**Turkey and Spinach Stuffed Sweet Potatoes**

*Serves*: 2

*Preparation Time*: 35 minutes

**Ingredients:**

- 2 medium sweet potatoes, scrubbed
- 4 oz lean ground turkey
- 1 cup fresh spinach, chopped
- 1 tablespoon olive oil
- 1 teaspoon smoked paprika
- 1 teaspoon garlic powder

**Instructions:**

1. Preheat the oven to 400°F, pierce sweet potatoes with a fork, and bake for 25–30 minutes until tender.
2. Cook ground turkey in olive oil until browned, then add spinach and cook until wilted. Season with smoked paprika and garlic powder.
3. Slice sweet potatoes, mash slightly, and fill with turkey and spinach mixture.
4. Serve warm and enjoy this hearty, nutrient-rich meal.

## **Why It's Good for AFib:**

Sweet potatoes are high in potassium, which supports a healthy heart rhythm. The lean turkey and spinach add protein, magnesium, and vitamins, making this meal a filling and heart-friendly option.

# Heart-Healthy Snacks: Quick Bites for Energy & Stability

**Apple Slices with Almond Butter**

**Ingredients:**

- 1 medium apple, sliced
- 1–2 tablespoons almond butter

**Instructions:**

Spread almond butter on each apple slice and enjoy!

**Why It's Good for AFib**

This snack is a natural source of potassium and healthy fats, keeping your blood sugar and heart rhythm steady.

## Trail Mix (Homemade, No Salt)

### Ingredients:

- ¼ cup unsalted almonds
- ¼ cup walnuts
- 2 tablespoons dried cranberries
- 1 tablespoon sunflower seeds

### Instructions:

Combine all ingredients in a small bowl or container for a portable, energy-boosting snack.

### Why It's Good for AFib

The mix provides magnesium, omega-3s, and fiber while avoiding excess sodium or sugar found in store-bought mixes.

**Rice Cakes with Avocado**

**Ingredients:**

- 1 plain, unsalted rice cake
- ¼ ripe avocado
- A dash of lemon juice

**Instructions:**

1. Mash the avocado in a small bowl.
2. Spread it over the rice cake.
3. Add a squeeze of lemon juice on top for extra flavor.

**Why It's Good for AFib:**

This snack gives you healthy fats and potassium from the avocado, both of which are good for your heart. The rice cake provides a light base without any added salt.

**Plain Popcorn with Olive Oil**

**Ingredients:**

- 2 cups plain, air-popped popcorn
- 1 teaspoon olive oil
- A pinch of garlic powder or paprika (optional)

**Instructions:**

1. Drizzle olive oil over the popcorn and toss it gently to coat.
2. Sprinkle a little garlic powder or paprika if you want extra flavor.

**Why It's Good for AFib:**

Popcorn is a whole grain that adds fiber to your diet, and olive oil provides heart-healthy fats. This snack is light, low in sodium, and easy to make!

# Desserts: Sweet Treats Without the Sugar Overload

**Baked Cinnamon Pears**

*Serves*: 2

*Preparation Time*: 25 minutes

**Ingredients:**

- 2 ripe pears, halved and cored
- ½ teaspoon cinnamon
- 1 teaspoon honey or maple syrup
- 1 tablespoon chopped walnuts

**Instructions:**

1. Preheat the oven to 375°F (190°C). Place the pear halves on a baking sheet, cut side up.
2. Sprinkle each pear with cinnamon and drizzle a little honey or maple syrup on top.
3. Bake for 20–25 minutes, until tender and slightly caramelized.
4. Top with a few chopped walnuts for a bit of crunch.

**Why It's Good for AFib**

The natural sweetness of pears and cinnamon satisfies cravings without processed sugar, while the walnuts add omega-3s and flavor.

## Greek Yogurt and Berry Parfait

*Serves*: 1

*Preparation Time*: 5 minutes

### Ingredients:

- ½ cup plain low-fat Greek yogurt
- ½ cup mixed berries (blueberries, strawberries, raspberries)
- 1 teaspoon flaxseeds or chia seeds

### Instructions:

1. Layer yogurt and berries in a small glass. Sprinkle flaxseeds on top.
2. Serve as a refreshing and heart-healthy dessert.

### Why It's Good for AFib

This dessert combines probiotics from the yogurt with antioxidants and fiber from the berries, promoting gut and heart health.

## Chocolate Banana "Nice" Cream

*Serves*: 2

*Preparation Time*: 10 minutes (plus 2 hours freezing time)

### Ingredients:

- 2 ripe bananas, sliced and frozen
- 1 tablespoon unsweetened cocoa powder
- 1 teaspoon almond butter (optional)

### Instructions:

1. Place the frozen banana slices in a blender or food processor.
2. Add the cocoa powder and almond butter if using. Blend until creamy, stopping to scrape down the sides as needed.
3. Serve immediately for a soft-serve texture or freeze for an additional hour if you prefer a firmer consistency.

### Why It's Good for AFib:

Bananas are a great source of potassium, which helps with heart rhythm stability, while the unsweetened cocoa powder adds antioxidants without excess sugar. This dessert satisfies your sweet tooth in a heart-healthy way.

## Baked Apple with Oats and Almonds

*Serves*: 1

*Preparation Time*: 10 minutes

### Ingredients:

- 1 medium apple, cored
- 1 tablespoon rolled oats
- 1 teaspoon almond slivers
- ½ teaspoon cinnamon
- 1 teaspoon honey or maple syrup
- 1 tablespoon water

### Instructions:

1. Preheat the oven to 375°F (190°C).
2. Place the apple in a small ovenproof dish. Stuff the center with oats, almonds, and cinnamon.
3. Drizzle honey or maple syrup over the filled apple. Add the water to the bottom of the dish to prevent drying.
4. Bake for 30 minutes, or until the apple is soft and the filling is golden.
5. Allow to cool slightly and enjoy warm.

### Why It's Good for AFib:

Apples provide natural sweetness and fiber, while oats and almonds contribute heart-healthy nutrients like magnesium and beneficial fats. The gentle sweetness of this dessert makes it a satisfying, guilt-free option.

These recipes are designed to give you heart-friendly, satisfying options for every part of your day. Whether it's a quick breakfast, a comforting dinner, or a sweet snack, you'll have the tools to enjoy meals while staying mindful of your AFib management goals. Now, enjoy cooking up your new favorites!

# The 3-Week AFib Action Plan for Seniors

Managing atrial fibrillation (AFib) can feel overwhelming, but taking it step by step makes all the difference. This 3-week action plan is here to guide you, focusing on small changes, sustainable routines, and long-term habits for heart health. Below, you'll find detailed daily instructions to make positive changes at a pace that's practical and achievable.

## Week 1: Small Tweaks for Big Impact

Week 1 is all about making small, focused changes that can make a meaningful difference in your heart health. By prioritizing hydration, reducing processed foods, and identifying what might be triggering your AFib, you'll set the groundwork for long-term success. Each day includes manageable steps to help you ease into these adjustments with confidence.

**Day 1 - Focus on Hydration**

**Action Plan:**

- Aim to drink at least 8-10 glasses of water throughout the day. Use a bottle or glass that helps you measure your intake and keep it nearby as a visual reminder.
- Replace one sugary or caffeinated drink (coffee, soda, sweet tea, etc.) with water, herbal tea, or infused water (try adding fresh lemon or cucumber slices).
- Track how much water you're drinking and note how you feel by the end of the day. Are you less tired?

**Why It Matters:** Dehydration can strain your heart, sometimes worsening symptoms like palpitations or dizziness. By staying hydrated, you'll give your heart the support it needs to function efficiently. Plus, reducing sugary drinks helps lower inflammation over time.

## Day 2 - Start a Food Journal
### Action Plan:

- Write down everything you eat and drink today. Include the time, portion sizes, and how you're feeling afterward (for example, "dizzy 30 minutes after lunch" or "no symptoms after snack").
- Pay extra attention to meals or snacks that might include processed foods, like chips, frozen dishes, or packaged bread.

**Why It Matters:** Keeping a food journal helps you spot patterns that might not be obvious right away. Processed foods, for example, are often high in sodium or additives that could trigger symptoms. Reflecting on your eating habits without judgment lays the foundation for gradual improvement.

**Tips for Success:** If writing down your meals feels like a hassle, use a simple checklist in your phone or keep a printed chart on your kitchen counter to make it easier.

**Day 3 - Begin with a Heart-Friendly Breakfast**

**Action Plan:**

- Choose one of these simple, nutritious breakfasts:
    - ***Oatmeal Bowl***: Top plain oatmeal with fresh berries, a sprinkle of nuts, and a drizzle of honey.
    - ***Power Scramble***: Whisk eggs with spinach or tomato slices, served with whole-grain toast.
    - ***Morning Smoothie***: Blend unsweetened yogurt, frozen berries, and a handful of spinach for a quick, on-the-go option.
- Avoid processed cereals or pastries that are often loaded with added sugars.

**Why It Matters:** A balanced breakfast can stabilize your blood sugar and reduce any afternoon cravings for less healthy choices. Eating nutrient-rich whole foods helps you feel energized and gives your heart the nutrients it needs to thrive.

## Day 4 - Be Mindful of Sodium Levels

**Action Plan:**

- Take a moment today to read the nutrition labels on the foods you eat or have stored in your pantry.
- Pay particular attention to the sodium content in items like canned soups, dressings, bread, and frozen meals.
- Whenever possible, opt for low-sodium alternatives to make healthier choices.
- Cook one meal from scratch using natural flavors instead of salt. For example:
  - ***Herb-Roasted Vegetables***: Season zucchini, bell peppers, and carrots with olive oil, rosemary, and garlic.
  - ***Simple Lemon Chicken***: Marinate chicken breast with lemon juice, pepper, and fresh parsley before baking.
- Avoid sprinkling extra salt at the table. Use flavorful spices instead, such as paprika, cumin, or basil.

**Why It Matters:** High sodium levels can lead to fluid retention and increased blood pressure, which can trigger AFib episodes. By reducing sodium, you're keeping stress off your heart.

## Day 5 - Identify Your Triggers

**Action Plan:** Review your food journal and reflect on your week so far. Have you noticed any foods or drinks that seem to make your symptoms worse? Common triggers include:

- Caffeine
- Alcohol
- Dehydration

Choose one suspected trigger to reduce for the rest of the week. For example, swap out your second cup of coffee for decaf or replace happy-hour cocktails with sparkling water.

**Why It Matters:** AFib triggers vary widely from person to person. Understanding your unique triggers puts you in control of your symptoms and empowers you to take preventive steps.

## Day 6 - Try Better Food Swaps

**Action Plan:**

- Make 2-3 swaps in your meals today. For example:
- Replace white rice with brown rice or quinoa.
- Ditch boxed mashed potatoes for roasted sweet potatoes.
- Use fresh lemon juice or balsamic vinegar instead of bottled dressings.
- During snack time, aim for whole, nutrient-dense options like:

- A handful of unsalted almonds.
- A piece of fruit like an apple or clementine.
- Greek yogurt with a sprinkle of cinnamon.

**Why It Matters:** Processed foods are often packed with added sugars, sodium, and unhealthy fats that can stress your heart. Even small swaps lead to big improvements in how your body processes food and maintains heart health.

**Day 7 - Review and Prep for Week 2**

**Action Plan:**

- Look back at your food journal and hydration logs. What changes made you feel better? Are there any habits that didn't work for you? Don't worry if not everything went perfectly—progress over perfection is the goal!
- Based on what you've learned, make a simple grocery list focusing on fresh produce, lean proteins, and whole grains.
- Take time to celebrate your success, whether it's drinking more water, reducing sodium, or discovering a new breakfast you love.

**Why It Matters:** Preparing for the week ahead prevents last-minute "what should I eat?" stress, making it easier to stay on track and keep building your healthy routine.

By the end of Week 1, you'll have built a foundation of positive habits you can continue to build upon. Even these small changes help you take control of your heart health and ease AFib symptoms. Celebrate each success, and get ready for Week 2 as your journey to long-term wellness continues!

## Week 2: Building a Sustainable Routine

With the small but meaningful changes you made in Week 1, you're ready to move into building a routine that works for your long-term heart health. Week 2 is all about introducing structure to your day-to-day habits so they become second nature.

You'll start meal prepping, focus on smarter grocery shopping, and actively track your symptoms to better understand what's working. This week is about creating a rhythm that supports your heart, energy levels, and overall well-being.

### Day 8 - Start Meal Planning

**Action Plan:** Take 15-20 minutes to plan your meals for the next 3-4 days. Keep it simple with basic components like:

- Lean proteins (chicken, fish, tofu, beans).
- Heart-friendly vegetables (spinach, bell peppers, carrots, broccoli).
- Whole grains (quinoa, brown rice, or 100% whole-wheat bread or pasta).

Ensure your plan includes a mix of meals you enjoy to avoid feeling deprived. For instance:

- A hearty vegetable soup for lunch.
- Grilled salmon with roasted sweet potatoes for dinner.
- A whole-grain muffin and a piece of fruit for breakfast.
- Double your portions when possible to save leftovers for the next day.

**Why It Matters:** Planned meals reduce the temptation of processed foods or last-minute unhealthy choices. Plus, cooking at home lets you control sodium and fat content. Consistency keeps you on track without having to think about "what's next."

## Day 9 - Shop Smart at the Grocery Store

**Action Plan:**

- Take your meal plan and create a grocery list. Organize it by sections of the store (produce, dairy, grains) to make shopping easier.
- Stick to the perimeter of the store where fresh foods like vegetables, lean meats, and dairy are usually found. Avoid the aisles with highly processed, packaged foods.

Read food labels carefully. Specifically, look for:

- Sodium content is lower than *140mg per serving*.
- No trans fats.

- Minimal added sugars (aim for less than 5*g per serving*).
- Try to include a rainbow of fruits and vegetables to give your heart a variety of nutrients.

**Why It Matters:** Smart grocery shopping is key to healthy eating. Having the right ingredients on hand makes it easier to prepare heart-friendly meals and avoid processed options.

## Day 10 - Prep Your Meals for the Week
**Action Plan:**

- Spend 30-45 minutes prepping food today. Focus on:
- Chopping vegetables so they're ready for cooking or snacking.
- Cooking grains in bulk, like brown rice or quinoa, to add to meals.
- Preparing one complete meal, like a stir-fry or roasted chicken with veggies. Store it in the fridge for an easy grab-and-heat option.
- Portioning out snacks into small containers or snack bags (e.g., almonds, baby carrots, or sliced cucumber).
- Label containers with dates so you know when to eat them.

**Why It Matters:** Prepping meals saves time and energy during the week, reducing the temptation to pick less healthy options. It's a simple way to stick to your plan, even on busy or low-energy days.

## Day 11 - Track Your Symptoms
### Action Plan:

- Use a small notebook or a tracking app to jot down how you're feeling today. Include:
- Any irregular heart rhythms or palpitations.
- Your energy levels (e.g., "felt tired after lunch").
- Anything new you tried in terms of food, hydration, or stress management.
- Be as specific as possible. For example, "Felt dizzy after eating frozen chicken pot pie" or "No symptoms after having oatmeal and berries for breakfast."
- Review at the end of the day for any potential patterns.

**Why It Matters:** Tracking symptoms helps you make informed decisions about what works for your body. Over time, you'll identify the best practices that keep your heart calm and steady.

## Day 12 - Rethink Your Snack Game
### Action Plan:

- Take stock of the snacks you're currently eating. Look for items that may be high in sodium, sugar, or unhealthy fats (e.g., chips, crackers, granola bars).
- Replace these with whole, nutrient-dense options like:
- A handful of unsalted nuts (e.g., almonds, walnuts).

- Fresh fruit (e.g., apple slices, orange segments, or grapes).
- Celery or carrot sticks with hummus.
- Prepare snacks ahead of time so they're easy to grab when you're hungry.

**Why It Matters:** Snack choices often sneak in unhealthy ingredients, but they're also an opportunity to add essential nutrients to your diet. Choosing the right snacks supports consistent energy levels and heart health.

## Day 13 - Reassess and Refresh

### Action Plan:

- Look at your food journal, symptom tracker, and meal plan so far this week. Reflect on:
- Which meals and snacks you enjoyed most.
- Whether you stayed hydrated and how it affected your symptoms.
- Any patterns between your symptoms and specific foods or habits.
- Adjust your grocery list or food prep plan as needed for next week. For instance, if brown rice feels heavy on your stomach, try quinoa instead. If a late-night snack causes discomfort, move it earlier in the evening.

**Why It Matters:** Building a sustainable routine requires flexibility. By tweaking your habits, you'll create a customized plan that feels natural and enjoyable.

### Day 14 - Reflect and Celebrate
### Action Plan:

- Reflect on how far you've come over the past two weeks. Write down or think about:
- What you've learned about your eating habits.
- Positive changes in how you feel physically or emotionally.
- Celebrate your success with a non-food reward. Treat yourself to something you enjoy, like a relaxing bath, a favorite movie, or a walk outdoors.
- Prepare for Week 3 by setting a simple goal, such as increasing daily movement or trying a new heart-healthy recipe.

**Why It Matters:** Celebrating your progress is essential for staying motivated. Recognizing small wins builds confidence and helps you stay committed to your long-term goals.

By the end of Week 2, you'll have established a routine that sets you up for success every day. From smart grocery shopping to symptom tracking, these steps make healthy living easier and more effective. Get ready to build on these habits in Week 3 as you focus on movement, stress management, and strengthening connections!

# Week 3: Lifestyle Habits for Long-Term Heart Health

With two weeks of groundwork in place, Week 3 focuses on habits that will sustain your progress and continue to benefit your heart in the long run. This week centers on gentle exercise, managing stress, and cultivating social connections.

These habits not only bolster your physical health but also positively influence your emotional and mental well-being. Each day provides simple, actionable steps to integrate these practices into your life.

**Day 15 - Start Moving with Gentle Activity.**

**Action Plan:**

- Begin with 10-15 minutes of low-impact exercise. Options include:
- A relaxed walk around your block or local park.
- Simple chair exercises, such as leg lifts or seated arm stretches.
- Beginner yoga, focusing on gentle poses or stretches (many online videos cater to seniors).
- Pay attention to your breathing and heart rate. Movement should feel comfortable and not overly tiring.

If you're using any heart-monitoring devices, jot down how your heart responds to the activity to track your progress over time.

**Why It Matters:** Regular movement strengthens your heart and circulation without overloading your system. Gentle, consistent exercise reduces the risk of future AFib episodes.

### Day 16 - Practice Deep Breathing to Reduce Stress

**Action Plan:** Set aside two 5-minute sessions for deep-breathing exercises, once in the morning and once in the evening. A simple technique is the **4-4-6 Method**:

- Breathe in through your nose for 4 seconds.
- Hold your breath for 4 seconds.
- Exhale slowly through your mouth for 6 seconds.
- Repeat for the full 5 minutes.

Find a quiet space where you can sit comfortably, focusing solely on your breath.

Explore other options if deep breathing isn't your favorite. Gentle music, meditation apps, or even a calming hobby like knitting can serve as stress relievers.

**Why It Matters:** Stress is a known AFib trigger, as it increases inflammation and puts pressure on your heart. Deep breathing signals your body to relax, bringing down your heart rate and helping you feel at ease.

## Day 17 - Nurture Social Connections

**Action Plan:** Reach out to one friend, family member, or neighbor for a chat. This could be a phone call, a short visit, or even a video call if you're far away.

- Plan a simple activity to do with someone, such as:
- Taking a short walk together.
- Sharing a meal or coffee (choose heart-friendly options!).
- Playing a favorite board or card game.

If you feel isolated, look for local senior groups, AFib support groups, or community activities where you can meet others with similar experiences.

**Why It Matters:** Strong social connections reduce stress, which is good for your heart and overall well-being. Spending time with loved ones or peers can help you feel supported, hopeful, and motivated to stick with healthy habits.

## Day 18 - Extend Your Gentle Exercise Routine

**Action Plan:** Add 5 extra minutes to the activity you started earlier this week, making it a 15-20 minute routine. Listen to your body and stop if you feel tired or faint.

- Try introducing variety to maintain interest, such as:
- Gardening or light yardwork.
- Stretching routines or tai chi, which are low impact and great for balance.

- Dancing to your favorite music in the living room.
- Continue monitoring your heart rate and energy levels during and after these activities.

**Why It Matters:** Increasing your physical activity steadily improves cardiovascular fitness without overexerting your heart. A little more movement each day helps tone muscles, ease stress, and boost endorphins, which make you feel good.

**Day 19 - Simplify and Minimize Stress in Daily Life**

**Action Plan:** Identify one task, commitment, or activity that feels unnecessarily stressful. Delegate it, postpone it, or remove it from your schedule entirely.

- Set aside 10-15 minutes for something purely enjoyable and relaxing, such as:
- Reading a favorite book or magazine.
- Listening to soothing music.
- Spending time with a pet.

Avoid multitasking today. Practice focusing on one thing at a time to help your mind and body feel balanced.

**Why It Matters:** Daily stressors can contribute to AFib symptoms, as stress triggers the release of hormones like adrenaline. Finding ways to simplify your day minimizes this burden, giving your heart and mind much-needed rest.

## Day 20 - Build Community and Share Meals
### Action Plan:

- Invite a friend, family member, or neighbor over for a meal. Choose a heart-healthy menu together, such as baked fish, steamed vegetables, and a fruit dessert.
- If you prefer eating out, pick a restaurant that offers menu options with fresh, whole ingredients and lower sodium.
- Focus on eating mindfully during the meal. Put away distractions, chew slowly, and savor each bite.

**Why It Matters:** Eating together encourages slower, more conscious meals that are better for digestion. It also helps create strong social bonds, which are essential for emotional and physical health.

## Day 21 - Reflect and Set Future Goals

**Action Plan:** Write down three things you're proud of from the past three weeks. Examples might include:

- Drinking more water daily.
- Trying a new vegetable or recipe.
- Feeling more energetic because of better food and exercise habits.

Set one or two small goals for the next month to continue your momentum. These might include:

- Walking for 20 minutes every day.
- Experimenting with three new low-sodium recipes.
- Scheduling regular check-ins with a friend or family member.
- Celebrate your success with a treat that supports your spirit and health, such as a new cozy sweater for walks, a yoga class, or a bouquet of fresh flowers.

**Why It Matters:** Reflecting on your progress helps you see how far you've come and motivates you to keep going. Setting new goals keeps your health plan fresh and engaging.

By completing Week 3, you've solidified habits that nurture your heart and support your overall well-being. Gentle exercise, stress management, and fostering social connections address not only your AFib but your whole self.

Remember, a healthy lifestyle is a lifelong commitment, but you now have the tools and foundation to continue your progress. Celebrate this milestone and look forward to all that a healthier heart will bring!

# Beyond Diet – Lifestyle Tips for Senior AFib Management

While diet is a critical component of managing AFib, it's not the whole picture. A healthy lifestyle that addresses emotional well-being, physical activity, sleep, and effective communication with healthcare providers can significantly improve heart health and quality of life. This chapter explores these aspects, offering practical tips tailored specifically for seniors.

## Managing Stress and Anxiety for a Calmer Heart

Stress and anxiety can wreak havoc on your heart, often triggering or worsening AFib symptoms. Stress-related hormones like adrenaline can disrupt your heart's rhythm, leading to uncomfortable episodes. Finding ways to manage stress is particularly important as a senior, as your body may not recover from stressors as quickly as it once did.

Here are some practical strategies to help you keep calm and steady your heart:

- *Mindfulness and Meditation*: Simple mindfulness practices, like focusing on your breath or observing your surroundings without judgment, can reduce stress. Guided meditations or apps specifically designed for relaxation may also help. Start with just five minutes a day and build up as you feel comfortable.
- *Deep Breathing Exercises*: When you're feeling anxious, deep breathing can calm your nervous system. Try this simple exercise: Breathe in slowly through your nose for a count of four, hold the breath for four counts, and exhale through your mouth for a count of six. Repeat this for a few minutes to feel more centered.
- *Engage in Hobbies*: Doing something you enjoy is a great stress reliever. Whether it's gardening, knitting, painting, or even birdwatching, hobbies can keep your mind engaged and your heart calm.
- *Gentle Socializing*: Connecting with others can help reduce feelings of isolation and anxiety. Whether it's talking to a friend on the phone, attending a community center event, or joining a support group for seniors with AFib, staying socially active can do wonders for your emotional health.
- *Limit Stress Triggers*: Identify specific situations or habits that cause you stress. It could be watching too much upsetting news, overcommitting to events, or

rushing through the day without breaks. Once you know your triggers, you can find ways to avoid or manage them.

Managing stress and anxiety is key to supporting a healthier heart and reducing AFib symptoms. By incorporating simple strategies like mindfulness, deep breathing, and engaging in enjoyable activities, you can create a calmer, more balanced lifestyle.

# The Role of Light Exercise and Safe Physical Activity

Light, low-impact exercise is great for seniors with atrial fibrillation (AFib) as it improves circulation, strengthens the heart, and reduces stress. However, it's important to avoid overexertion to prevent triggering symptoms. This section covers the benefits of gentle activity, examples of heart-healthy exercises, and tips to get started safely.

### Why Light Exercise Matters for Seniors with AFib

Exercise offers many benefits, but for seniors, light and moderate activities are ideal. Here's why exercise is essential for heart health and overall well-being in older adults with AFib:

- ***Improves Circulation***: Movement helps oxygen-rich blood flow more efficiently through your body, which can reduce strain on the heart.

- ***Strengthens the Heart Muscle***: Engaging in safe physical activity can help your heart pump blood more effectively, potentially making it less prone to irregular rhythms.
- ***Lowers Blood Pressure***: Many gentle exercises help reduce high blood pressure, which is a significant risk factor for AFib.
- ***Reduces Stress***: Light activities like walking or yoga can naturally lower stress hormones like cortisol, which can trigger AFib episodes.
- ***Supports Weight Maintenance***: Regular movement helps manage weight, easing physical stress on the heart.
- ***Improves Mobility and Balance***: Keeping active strengthens your muscles and joints, enhancing your balance and reducing the risk of falls. This is vital for seniors who may struggle with other health concerns like arthritis or joint pain.

By prioritizing low-impact activities suited to your abilities, you can enjoy these benefits without overstressing your body.

**Safe and Effective Exercises for Seniors**

For seniors with AFib, it's essential to choose exercises designed to be kind to the joints, low intensity, and focused on maintaining balance and strength. Below are some excellent options to explore:

1. ***Walking***: Walking is one of the simplest and most effective forms of exercise for heart health. It's accessible, requires no equipment besides a comfortable pair of shoes, and can be done almost anywhere.

   **<u>Why It Works:</u>**

   Walking at a steady, moderate pace gets your heart rate up without overexerting your cardiovascular system. It also strengthens your leg muscles, improves circulation, and helps reduce high blood pressure.

   **<u>How to Make It Safe and Enjoyable:</u>**

   - Start with short walks of 10-15 minutes a day, gradually increasing to 20-30 minutes as your stamina improves.
   - Choose flat, even surfaces like sidewalks, parks, or indoor tracks to minimize the risk of tripping.
   - Wear supportive shoes that fit well and provide cushioning for your feet and joints.
   - Walk with a friend or family member if you enjoy company, or listen to calming music to motivate yourself.
2. ***Chair Yoga or Gentle Yoga***: Yoga can be incredibly beneficial for older adults by improving flexibility, stability, and relaxation. Chair yoga is a modified

version designed for seniors who prefer a seated option, eliminating the need to get on and off the floor.

**Why It Works:**

Yoga focuses on gentle stretches and deep breathing, promoting relaxation and improving blood flow. These benefits can calm your heart rate, reduce stress, and enhance joint mobility.

**How to Get Started Safely:**

- Join a yoga class that caters specifically to seniors or AFib patients, often available at community centers or yoga studios.
- Follow video tutorials for chair yoga sessions in the comfort of your home.
- Avoid poses that require extended periods of bending or holding your breath, as these could put extra strain on your heart.
- Always listen to your body; pause if you feel any discomfort or dizziness.

3. *Water Aerobics*: Water-based exercise provides a low-impact environment, making it particularly helpful for those with arthritis or joint pain. Exercises performed in the water minimize strain on your body while still improving heart health and overall fitness.

**Why It Works:**

Water's buoyancy reduces the impact on joints, allowing you to move freely without pain. Meanwhile, the resistance of the water adds gentle strength training benefits.

**How to Participate Safely:**

- Look for senior-focused water aerobics classes, which are often shorter and less intense.
- Start slow with basic movements like leg lifts or gentle arm sweeps to gauge how your body responds.
- Use the pool's railing for balance when needed, and opt for shallow water if deep water feels unsafe.
- Stay hydrated, as the water can make you feel less thirsty even though you're exercising.

4. *Tai Chi*: Tai Chi is an ancient Chinese practice that consists of slow, graceful movements combined with focused breathing. It's known for improving balance, flexibility, and mental clarity, making it an excellent option for seniors managing AFib.

**Why It Works:**

The gentle, flowing movements of Tai Chi promote relaxation and reduce stress, both of which can help stabilize your heart rhythm. It's also great for improving coordination and preventing falls.

### How to Get a Good Start:

- Join a beginner-level Tai Chi class at a senior center or community program.
- Practice in an open, uncluttered area to avoid tripping hazards.
- Focus on your breathing as you move; this can help regulate your heart rate and instill a sense of calm.

**Practical Tips for Safe Exercise for Seniors**

Whether you're new to exercise or returning after some time off, safety should always come first. Follow these tips to build a sustainable routine:

1. *Consult Your Doctor*: Before beginning any new activity, speak with your healthcare provider. They can guide you on the right intensity level, recommend specific exercises, or identify any precautions based on your current medications and health status.
2. *Start Slow and Gradual*: If you haven't been active in a while, start with just a few minutes per day and gradually increase the duration. Listen to your body and stop if you experience dizziness, shortness of breath, or palpitations.
3. *Warm Up and Cool Down*: Warming up before exercise helps prepare your body, while cooling down

afterward prevents cramps or sudden drops in blood pressure. Gentle stretches work well for both purposes.
4. ***Stay Hydrated***: Seniors are more susceptible to dehydration, which can trigger AFib. Drink water before, during, and after exercise to keep your body replenished.
5. ***Consider Your Surroundings***: Choose environments that minimize fall risks, such as paved trails, well-lit gyms, or the inside of your home.
6. ***Use Assistive Devices if Needed***: If balance or joint pain is a concern, don't hesitate to use canes, walk tracks, or chairs during exercise.
7. ***Mix It Up***: Keep your routine interesting by combining different activities like walking one day and Tai Chi the next. This variety improves overall fitness and keeps you motivated.

By incorporating these light but impactful exercises into your routine, you can empower yourself to strengthen your heart, improve your mobility, and enjoy better overall health. Remember, the key is consistency and listening to your body so you can move safely and confidently towards better well-being.

# Sleep and AFib: How to Improve Rest as You Age

A good night's sleep is essential for everyone, but it's especially important if you're managing AFib. Poor sleep can increase stress hormones, worsen heart rhythms, and make AFib symptoms harder to manage. Many seniors struggle with sleep issues, such as insomnia or sleep apnea, but small changes in your routine can make a big difference.

Here's how to prioritize better sleep for your heart health:

- *Create a Sleep-Friendly Environment*: Ensure your bedroom is quiet, dark, and cool. Using blackout curtains or a white noise machine can help block disturbances that might wake you up.
- *Stick to a Sleep Schedule*: Going to bed and waking up at the same time every day, even on weekends, can regulate your body's internal clock and make it easier to fall and stay asleep.
- *Limit Screen Time Before Bed*: Bright screens from phones, tablets, or TVs can disrupt your body's natural sleep signals. Try shutting off devices at least an hour before bed and engaging in relaxing activities like reading or meditating instead.
- *Address Sleep Apnea or Other Issues*: Sleep apnea, a condition where breathing briefly stops during sleep, is common among seniors and can worsen AFib. If you snore heavily or often feel tired during the day despite

sleeping, discuss this with your doctor to explore treatment options.
- ***Avoid Sleep Disruptors***: Cut back on caffeine or alcohol in the hours leading up to bed and keep heavy meals or exercise earlier in the day.

Prioritizing quality sleep is crucial for managing AFib and supporting overall heart health. By making small, consistent changes to your sleep habits, you can improve your rest and better manage your symptoms as you age.

## How to Talk to Your Doctor About Diet and Medication Interactions

Your healthcare provider is a key partner in managing AFib, and clear communication is crucial for tailoring the best plan for you. Medications can come with side effects or dietary restrictions, so discussing your diet and lifestyle is essential to avoid potential problems.

Here are tips to make the most of your appointments:

- ***Prepare Questions in Advance***: Write down specific questions about your medication and diet so you don't forget during the appointment. For example, you might ask, "Are there any foods I should avoid while taking these medications?" or "Does weight loss from dietary changes affect my dosage?"

- ***Bring a List of Medications***: Include all prescriptions, supplements, and over-the-counter medications you're taking. Some supplements, like fish oil or vitamin K, can interact with blood thinners or other heart medications.
- ***Track Symptoms and Share Them***: Keep a diary of your symptoms, dietary changes, and physical activity. This information can help your doctor fine-tune your treatment plan.
- ***Ask About Monitoring***: Some seniors with AFib may benefit from periodic blood tests to evaluate the effectiveness of their medications and check for potential nutrient deficiencies. Discuss whether this is necessary for you.
- ***Be Honest About Your Lifestyle***: Your doctor can only provide the best advice if they have a clear picture of your habits, struggles, and overall health.

Taking the time to build an open dialogue with your doctor can prevent complications and give you more confidence in managing your condition.

By tackling stress, incorporating light physical activities, improving your sleep, and maintaining open communication with your healthcare provider, you're addressing major lifestyle factors that influence AFib. These changes, combined with an AFib-friendly diet, can help you take control of your heart health and enjoy a more active, fulfilling life.

# **Conclusion**

You've come so far in understanding how to take control of your heart health, and this is just the beginning of a positive, empowered chapter in your life. Staying consistent with dietary and lifestyle changes is entirely within your reach when you take things slowly and focus on small, meaningful steps.

Don't try to take on everything at once; instead, make one change and give yourself time to adjust. When a new habit begins to feel natural, move on to another. Celebrate your progress, no matter how small, because each step is a testament to your commitment to a healthier, stronger heart. If you ever feel overwhelmed, remind yourself that it's about steady improvement, not perfection.

Your heart health can benefit from small adjustments that fit seamlessly into your everyday life. Choosing meals that are both simple and nourishing, preparing food in advance to save time and effort, and drinking plenty of water throughout the day are all little things that have a big impact when done consistently.

Gentle movement, like a daily walk or trying out a calming activity like Tai Chi, can also strengthen your heart and keep your body energized. By focusing on ease and enjoyment, these changes become part of your routine without feeling like a burden.

You don't have to go through this alone. There are so many ways to find support and connection. Online communities are a valuable way to meet others who understand what it's like to manage AFib.

If you prefer in-person interaction, check out local senior centers, libraries, or community organizations that offer wellness classes or health education events. Reaching out to your doctor or healthcare provider is another way to get answers and reassurance if you have questions or concerns. Surrounding yourself with a network of supportive people can make the path ahead feel less uncertain and more manageable.

The steps you take today can shape a healthier, brighter tomorrow. With the knowledge and tools you now have, you're in control of your heart's well-being. By leaning on the support around you and staying committed to practical, achievable changes, you're setting yourself up for a life full of energy, resilience, and a deep sense of accomplishment.

# FAQs

**What foods should I avoid if I have AFib?**

Avoid foods high in sodium, trans fats, and added sugar. This includes processed snacks, canned soups, fast food, fried items, and sugary beverages. Limiting alcohol and caffeine is also a good idea, as they can trigger irregular heart rhythms.

**Are there any specific nutrients I should focus on?**

Yes! Aim for foods rich in potassium, magnesium, and omega-3 fatty acids, like bananas, leafy greens, salmon, and walnuts. These nutrients help maintain a healthy heart rhythm and reduce inflammation.

**Can I make heart-healthy meals on a budget?**

Absolutely! Choose affordable, nutrient-dense options like dried lentils, oats, frozen vegetables, and canned fish (in water, with no added salt). These are budget-friendly and versatile for meal preparation.

**How can I reduce sodium when cooking?**

Use fresh herbs, spices, lemon juice, or garlic for flavor instead of salt. Look for "low-sodium" or "no-salt-added" products, and avoid pre-packaged spice mixes that often contain hidden salt.

**Is it okay to snack, and what are the best snack options for AFib?**

Snacks are fine as long as they're healthy and balanced. Great options include unsalted nuts, fresh fruit with nut butter, plain yogurt with berries, or raw veggie sticks with hummus. These snacks provide nutrients without adding excess sodium or sugar.

**Should I completely avoid caffeine?**

Not necessarily. Some people with AFib can tolerate moderate amounts of caffeine, such as a cup of coffee, green tea, or other caffeinated beverages, without experiencing any issues. In fact, research suggests that low to moderate caffeine intake may not significantly increase the risk of triggering symptoms for everyone.

However, it's important to listen to your body, as caffeine sensitivity varies from person to person. If you notice that caffeine seems to trigger symptoms like heart palpitations or discomfort, it's best to limit your intake and consult your doctor to determine what's safe for you.

**How can I ensure I'm eating enough while managing AFib?**

Focus on smaller, well-balanced meals throughout the day. Include lean proteins, whole grains, and plenty of fruits and vegetables to meet your energy and nutritional needs. If you're unsure, consider working with a registered dietitian for personalized guidance.

# References and Helpful Links

Morales-Brown, L. (2024, February 14). What is the best AFib diet? https://www.medicalnewstoday.com/articles/afib-diet

Britt, T. (2024, April 19). Treating atrial fibrillation in older individuals. https://www.medicalnewstoday.com/articles/atrial-fibrillation-treatment-in-elderly

Does older age increase the risk of atrial fibrillation? (n.d.). Mayo Clinic. https://www.mayoclinic.org/diseases-conditions/atrial-fibrillation/expert-answers/atrial-fibrillation-age-risk/faq-20118478

Atrial fibrillation - Symptoms and causes. (n.d.). Mayo Clinic. https://www.mayoclinic.org/diseases-conditions/atrial-fibrillation/symptoms-causes/syc-20350624

Aging changes in the heart and blood vessels: MedlinePlus Medical Encyclopedia. (n.d.). https://medlineplus.gov/ency/article/004006.htm

Volgman, A. S., Nair, G., Lyubarova, R., Merchant, F. M., Mason, P., Curtis, A. B., Wenger, N. K., Aggarwal, N. T., Kirkpatrick, J. N., & Benjamin, E. J. (2022). Management of atrial fibrillation in patients 75 years and older. Journal of the American College of Cardiology, 79(2), 166–179. https://doi.org/10.1016/j.jacc.2021.10.037

Britt, T. (2024b, April 19). Treating atrial fibrillation in older individuals. https://www.medicalnewstoday.com/articles/atrial-fibrillation-treatment-in-elderly

www.ingramcontent.com/pod-product-compliance
Lightning Source LLC
LaVergne TN
LVHW012030060526
838201LV00061B/4547